DO IT YOURSELF BEFORE MEDICAL HELP ARRIVE.

(PART ONE)

HOW TO HANDLE EMERGENCY CONDITIONS

Clara Washington

Copyright © 2023

@Clara Washington

All rights reserved. No part of this book may be reproduced or transmitted in any form or by any means without written permission from the author. For further enquiry contact boundlessventures001@gmail.com

ISBN: XXXXXXXXXXXXX

INTRODUCTION

This book highlights some quick home remedy that can be administered to a person when an emergency occurs. The aim of this book is to help you take the correct action at the right time when faced with such an emergency, before proper medical help arrive. The author also identified what is wrong to do at that particular time, at the same time suggest the proper ways to handle such condition. This book is recommended for everyone because emergency Condition can happen to anybody at any time.

"A STITCH IN TIME SAVES NINE"

TABLE OF CONTENTS

1. BREATHING BLOCKAGE

2. BURNS

3. CHOKING

4. CONVULSION

5. DROWNING

6. FRACTURE

7. HEART ATTACK

8. POISON

9. CUT

10. NOSE BLEEDING

11. SNAKE BITE

12. SCORPION STING

DO IT YOURSELF BEFORE MEDICAL HELP ARRIVE.

(PART 1)

1. BREATHING BLOCKAGE: if someone had stopped breathing as a result of heart attack or food lodged in the air pipe. Use mouth-to-mouth resuscitation, otherwise known as the kiss of life, to bring back the victim to life. Steps:

(1) lay the victim face upwards.

(2) Loosen the clothing around the neck.

(3) Open the victim's mouth

(4) Take a deep breath, then place your mouth over the victim's mouth.

(5) give 4 or 5 full breaths into the victim's lungs.

(6) if the chest does not rise, then know that there is a blockage to the airflow. Repeat no. 4 again, until the victim start breathing or until medical help arrive.

2. BURNS: When someone is burned by a fire or a heat. The first thing to do is to try to relief the pains, before taking the person to the hospital for medical attention.

Steps to relive the pains are:

(1) Move the victim from the position of the flames immediately.

(2) Get a cool water or ice blocks and administer it to the affected area for some minutes.

(4) Allowed air to dry the area.

(5) Cover the burned area with a clean, dry cloth to prevent that area from being infected.

(6) Call for medical attention.

3. CHOKING: The most common cause of choking among children is when food lodge in the windpipe. That is why it is advisable for children not to talk while eating. Choking stop the victim from breathing, obviously because there is a blockage in the airways. Once that occurs, the person will be unable to speak.

Steps to remove the blockage from the child's throat are:

(1) Quickly hit the child on their neck, part of their shoulder.

(2) carry the child upside down or sit down and place the child over your kneels.

3) continue hitting the child on the back or neck part of the shoulder softly, (in an up side down position) until the object comes out.

(4) If the object did not come out, rush the child to the hospital immediately.

4. CONVULSION: Convulsion is often caused by illness such as high fever, poison, unstable body system, etc. among children or adults. It occurs suddenly. This will make the victim to collapse. Then the victim will start shaking violently.

(1) Hold the person and make him to lie on the ground face- uo.

(2) Once the victim stop shaking allow the victim to relax.

(3) Do not try to restrain the convulsion, rather loosen the victim cloth around the neck, chest, and waist in other to allow airflow.

(4) guarded him safely so that he will not injure himself during the seizure.

(5) Stay beside the victim until he wakes up.

(6) Advise him to go and see a doctor.

5. DROWNING : Drowning occurs when someone is suffocated in a sea, river, or in a swimming pool. When someone is drowned, water prevents the air from reaching the lungs. The steps to take in order to rescue the victim are :

(1) If you can swim or skilled in water rescue technique, try to pull the victim from the water immediately.

(2) Once you get the victim ashore, Lay the victim on the ground, faced up.

(3) Open the victim's nose and mouth, to ensure that the tongue or any object does not block the throat.

(4) apply artificial respiration (kiss of life).

(5) If the victim heart beat and breathing has stopped, give the victim heart massage.

(6) Repeat (3) & (4) until the victim's heart-beat and breathing have been restored.

(7) Then turn the victim to a recovery position (make him to lay on his stomach.

(8) Call for a medical assistant.

6. FRACTURE: Fracture occurs when someone has a hit, bruise or dislocation of the bones at the joint.

(1) Straighten the affected area.

(2) Tie a bandage (placed a padding) on the affected area.

(3) Take the victim to the hospital.

7. HEART ATTACK: This often occurs when there is reduced blood supply to the muscles of the heart, resulting from a blockage of the coronary arteries.

When someone has a heart attack

(1) Move the victim as quick and gently as possible.

(1) Hold the victim and place him in a comfortable position.

(2) Let the victim be in a sitting position with the back well-supported.

(4) feel the victim's heart beats, whether it have stopped.

(3) Make sure that the sitting position which you placed the victim does not interfere with blood circulation.

(4) If the victim heart has stopped beating, lay the victim on the floor, face-up, start heart massage at once.

(6) Call for medical assistant immediately.

Note: do not apply heart massage if the person's heart is still beating.

8. POISON: Poison can be eaten, drink, or inhaled. When someone drank or ate a poisonous substance, the person should seek medical attention immediately. But before medical help arrive; steps can be taken to reduce the effect of the poison.

The Steps are:

(1) Give the victim plenty of water or milk to drink in order to dilute the poison.

(2) If the person is conscious, give him bitter-kola or garlic to chew, while waiting for medical attention. Natural Palm oil can also help to dilute the poison at the mean time.

(3) If the poison was inhaled by the victim, remove the victim from the place of poisoning immediately.

(4) If the person is unconscious, do not apply kiss of life or heart massage on him, rather take him to the hospital immediately.

9. CUT: cut occurs when a sharp blade penetrates the skin, allowing blood to flow out. When someone has a cut in the skin, the first thing to do is:

(1) Try to stop the bleeding, by apply firm pressure over the wound.

(2) If there is an object deep inside the wound, do not remove the object, bandage it, and take the victim to the hospital immediately.

(4) When bleeding stops. Wash the surface of the wound with water.

(5) Cover the wound with a clean cloth.

(6) Dry and cover the wound with a clean cloth.

(7) Apply a dressing over the cut.

(8) Take the victim to a nearby hospital or clinic for medical attention.

10. NOSE BLEEDING: Thus can occur as a result of a direct blow or injury to the nose. But sometimes nose bleed can occur without any obvious reason. In such a case, the person should be taken to a doctor immediately.

If the nose bleed is as a result of a direct blow on the nose,

(1) place the victim's head tilted forward over a sink or a bowl.

(2) Firmly pinch the nostrils until the bleeding stop.

(3) Tell the person to breathe through the mouth.

(4) Tell the person to avoid swallowing saliva at that moment.

(5) Apply an ice pack to the bridge of the nose and call for medical aid.

11. SNAKE BITES: This can occur when someone is bitten by a snake. Some snakes are very venomous, so when someone is bitten by them, the person should be taken to the hospital for medical attention immediately.

But some steps can be taken to reduce the effect of the venom before the person is taken to the hospital.

(1) Keep the bitten person still and calm.

(2) Get a strong rope and tie the area above the bitten wound, or use a tourniquet. This can slow down the spread of the venom.

(2) Use a sharp blade and cut the bitten wound, and attempt to suck out the venom with your mouth.

(3) Give the victim Bitter kola or Garlic to chew.

(4) Do not use ice pack on the victim.

(5) Do not give the victim water, alcohol are food to eat at that moment. In order to keep metabolism at low rate.

(6) Take the victim to the nearest hospital immediately.

12. SCORPION STING: Scorpion stings can be painful, but rarely life-threatening. It often causes swelling, redness, and burning sensation in the affected area. So, when someone is stung by a scorpion. Follow these steps to administer a quick remedy to it before taking the person to a nearby clinic for medical attention.

(1) Keep the victim still and clam.

(2) Clean the Sting surface.

(3) Apply fresh onion juice on the stung surface.

(4) The pains will subside immediately, then take the victim to a nearby hospital to see a doctor.

www.ingramcontent.com/pod-product-compliance
Lightning Source LLC
Chambersburg PA
CBHW050327220526
45465CB00005B/2174